Pit Boss Wood Pellet Grill & Smoker Cookbook 2021

A Tailor Made Program To Extra Juicy, Flavorful Summer Recipes For Beginners And Experts To Impress Your Friends And Become The Undisputed Pitmaster Of The Neighborhood

Steve R.Kendall

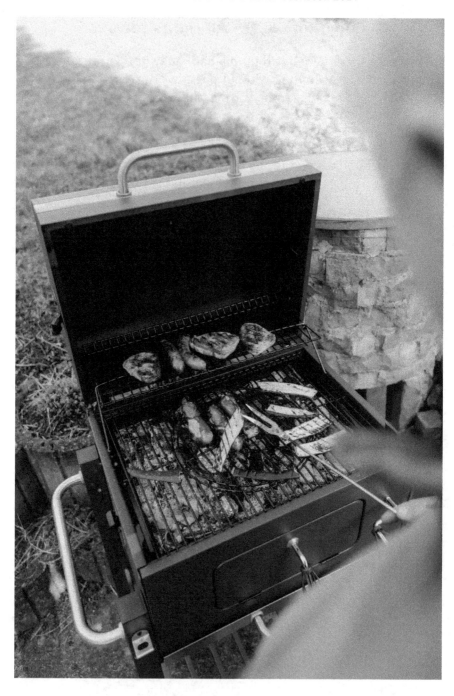

Table of Contents

INTRODUCTION 8

WHY A WOOD PELLET SMOKE AND GRILL? 12

WHAT IS A PELLET SMOKER AND GRILL? 13

WHY CHOOSE TO USE A WOOD PELLET SMOKER AND GRILL? 13

HOW TO USE A WOOD PELLET SMOKER AND GRILL? 14

WHAT DISHES CAN WE CAN ON A WOOD PELLET SMOKER AND GRILL? 14

ADVANTAGES OF WOOD PELLET SMOKER AND GRILL............................ 15

TEMPERATURE CONTROL 18

WHAT ARE THE PORTIONS OF A PELLET GRILL? 18

DIFFERENT TYPES FOR DIFFERENT MEAT FLAVORS............................... 23

FUNDAMENTALS OF WOOD PELLET COOKING 26

DIFFERENCE BETWEEN HOT AND COLD SMOKING................................ 28

APPETIZERS AND SIDES RECIPES 32

1.   BACON CHEDDAR SLIDER... 32

2.   APPLE WOOD SMOKED CHEESE.. 35

3.   HICKORY SMOKED MOINK BALL SKEWER 37

BEEF RECIPES 40

4.   ITALIAN BEEF SANDWICH... 40

5.   THAI BEEF SKEWERS 43

6.   BBQ CHILI BURGER 45

7.   TRAEGER FILET MIGNON 48

LAMP RECIPES 50

8.   GRILLED LAMB BURGERS WITH PICKLED ONIONS 50

9.   BRAISED LAMB SHANK 54

10. GREEK STYLE ROAST LEG OF LAMB RECIPE 56

11. SMOKED LAMB SAUSAGE 59

12. LAMB LOLLIPOPS WITH MANGO CHUTNEY 62

13. GRILLED LAMB CHOPS 65

CHICKEN RECIPES 68

14. SPICY BBQ CHICKEN 68

15. TRAEGER BBQ HALF CHICKENS 70

16. SMOKED DEVILED EGGS 72

17. PICKLED BRINED HOT CHICKEN SANDWICH 74

18. BAKED CHICKEN CORDON BLEU 78

TURKEY RECIPES 82

19. TURKEY JALAPENO MEATBALLS 82

20. WILD TURKEY SOUTHWEST EGG ROLLS 85

21. SMOKED WILD TURKEY BREAST 87

22. GRILLED WILD TURKEY ORANGE CASHEW SALAD 90

23. BAKED CORNBREAD TURKEY TAMALE PIE 93

24. BBQ PULLED TURKEY SANDWICHES 96

PORK RECIPES 98

25. ROSEMARY PORK TENDERLOIN 98

26. PULLED PORK 101

27. HONEY GLAZED HAM 104

28. SWEET & SALTY PORK BELLY 106

29. SWEET BACON WRAPPED SMOKES 108

30. PROSCIUTTO WRAPPED ASPARAGUS 110

31. LEMON PEPPER PORK TENDERLOIN 112

32. BACON WRAPPED JALAPENO POPPERS 114

33. PASTRAMI 116

34. BEEF JERKY 118

35. SMOKED BEEF ROAST 120

36. REVERSE SEARED FLANK STEAK 122

37. NEW YORK STRIP 124

SEAFOOD RECIPES 126

38. MARINATED HALIBUT STEAK IN GRAPEFRUIT JUICE 126

SAUCES 128

39. CHORAN SAUCE 128

40. HOT SAUCE WITH CILANTRO 129

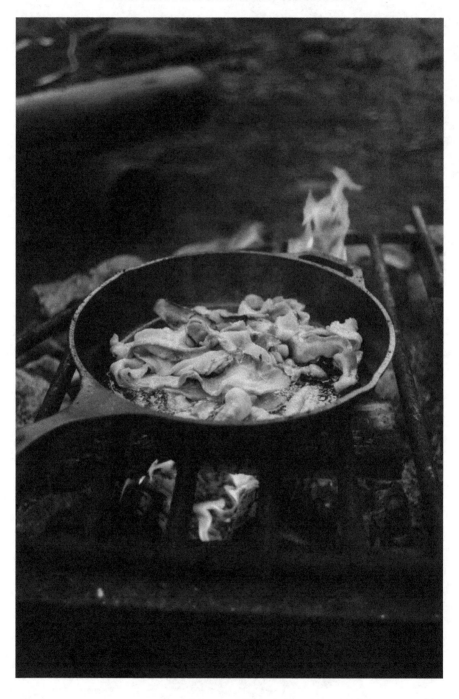

Introduction

This delicious cookbook is only for Food lovers. Do you want your favorite smoker grill recipes? Here is my cookbook which contains delicious and tasty smoke BBQ Grill recipes.

How Uo Use a Wood Pellet Smoker

The Wood Pellet Smoker-Grill utilizes wood pellets, which makes temperature and flavor control easier when smoking, grilling, or roasting. The ease of use has made this smoker-grill popular all around the globe.

Each Wood Pellet Smoker-Grill contains a storage hopper. This storage hopper is the place where you add all of the wood pellets. The equipment takes care of the transfer of wood pellets from the storage hopper to the burning area in the correct quantity.

Use of Different Wood Pellets In the Wood Pellet Smoke and Grill

Different types of wood pellets, such as apple, cherry, hickory, mesquite, and others, are used to obtain specific flavors in foods. Each type of wood pellet is considered suitable for certain types of foods. Knowing this is critically important so that you can get the best flavors out of your cooking.

1. Apple wood pellets are generally used when the food's main ingredient is pork, chicken, or vegetables.

2. Cherry wood pellets are perfect for baking food, including pork, lamb, chicken, and beef.

3. Hickory wood pellets make pork, beef, vegetables, and even poultry exceptionally delicious.

Along with these three types, there are other wood pellet options, such as alder, maple, mesquite, pecan, and oak. Pork dishes can get the best flavors with almost all kinds of wood pellets except oak and mesquite. Oak, alder, and mesquite types are more effective when you want to cook fish, shrimp, or other kinds of seafood.

The Wood Pellet Smoke and Grill is a durable and cost-effective option for anyone who wants to smoke or grill without worrying all the time. Because of its quality of construction, it works effectively for a long time. You only need to spend a few minutes after cooking to maintain its cleanliness. This keeps the fuel efficiency high and allows for controlled wood pellet burning.

History of the Wood Pellet Smoke and Grill

The very first Wood Pellet Smoker-Grill was introduced in 1985. Joe Traeger was the man behind the concept and the construction of the Wood Pellet Smoker-Grill. After spending a year creating his smoker-grill, he obtained a patent and started production at a commercial level. The smoker-grill looked similar to traditional smokers in terms of its exterior design. There was a drum barrel and a chimney. But the internal components were the true magic. Traeger divided the internal design into three parts. These three parts were the sections where wood pellets had to go in order to get burned.

The storage hopper was the first part, which worked as storage for the wood pellets in the smoker-grill. Then, the next stop for the pellets was the auger, which was a rotating section. This rotation allowed wood pellets to reach the third and final section. This final section was called a firebox or burning box. In this area, a fan allowed the proper distribution of the cultivated heat.

In the early designs, the user had to light the smoker-grill manually. However, the design got updated with time, and now, there are completely automatic Wood Pellet Smoker-Grills available.

The reduction in wood pellet size revolutionized the whole smoking and grilling process. The machine obtained the ability to balance the temperatures on its own for as long as required. This convenience wasn't available with charcoal burning smokers. At the same time, wood pellets also provided more variety based on the flavorful hardwood choices available.

That would not be wrong to say that the BBQ world experienced a revolution with the introduction of the Wood Pellet Smoker-Grill. Cooking got simpler and more comfortable, which gave even newbies a chance to smoke, grill, bake, and roast. The machine was capable of handling the temperature on its own, so the users could be stress-free and safe when cooking. In 2007, after the expiration of Traeger's patent, the Wood Pellet Smoker-Grill market opened for more advanced options. This led to more advancements and automation in the equipment.

Benefits of the Wood Pellet Smoker-Grill

1. Flavorful food

You work on your cooking techniques to get the best flavors possible. However, the techniques alone can't do it all. You need the right kind of equipment to get the correct flavor in your cooked dish. This is why the Wood Pellet Smoker-Grill is considered the best choice in the world of BBQ. The wood pellet flavors, such as cherry, apple, mesquite, and hickory, give different kinds of smoky flavors to the food. This flavor is way better than getting a charcoal aroma or a gaseous aroma when using other types of smokers. The natural flavor in your food enhances the deliciousness.

2. Ease of use

The modern-age designs of this smoker-grill alleviate all stress. You need to click a single button in order to begin the cooking process. The management of wood pellets happens is taken care of by the smoker, so you get the desired fire quality according to the kind of cooking process you want. Hence, barbeque becomes an easy task for everyone.

3. Different smoke temperatures

Since Wood Pellet Smoker-Grills can burn wood pellets in a variety of ways, you need different temperature levels for different processes. The smoke temperature options can range from 180°F to a maximum of 500°F. This wide temperature range makes one machine capable of all kinds of cooking, including smoking, grilling roasting, baking, and searing. You can pick any kind of meat and cook it to your desired level.

4. Temperature consistency

Unlike traditional smokers, Wood Pellet Smoker-Grills offer the consistent temperature you need for grilling or smoking. The wood pellets keep on reaching the burning section as required. This creates and maintains the same temperature during the whole cooking process.

Let's get to the recipes you can cook in your Wood Pellet Smoker-Grill!

WHY A WOOD PELLET SMOKE AND GRILL?

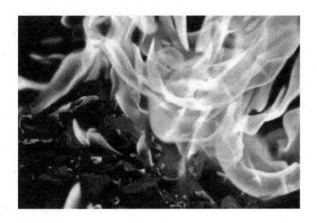

There is nothing more popular in the market nowadays than Pellet Smoker and Grills. And while a very few people claim that the popularity of pellet Smoker and Grill stems from its increase of use and the outstanding marketing for this product, the majority of people agree upon the fact that Pellet Smoker and Grills are acquiring its unrivaled popularity thanks to the effectiveness of this product.

Unlike any traditional grills people could have used in the past, Pellet Smoker and Grills are one of the most versatile, automated and perfect-to use revolutionary grills that one can rely on to get the flavor you dream of tasting. Pellet Smoker and Grills just make the perfect choice and the one and only best solution to cook any type of meat in a healthy way. Not only Pellet Smoker and Grills allow smoking ingredients, but it also allows a slow roasting process, baking a pizza or even perfectly grilling steak. However, this new revolutionary appliance is still not known by many people; so what is a Wood Pellet Smoker and Grill? So how can we use a Pellet Smoker and Grill?

What Is A Pellet Smoker And Grill?

To provide you with a clear answer about the Wood Pellet Smoker and Grill, let us start by defining this grilling appliance. In fact, Pellet Smoker and Grills can be defined as an electric outdoor Smoker and Grill that is only fueled by wood pellets. Wood Pellet is a type of fuel that is characterized by its capsule size and is praised for its ability to enhance more flavors and tastes to the chosen smoked meat. And what is unique and special about wood pellet as a fuel is that it can grill, smoke, roast, braise and even bake according is easily to follow instructions. I equipped with a control board that allows you to automatically maintain your desired temperature for several hours

Why Choose To Use A Wood Pellet Smoker And Grill?

The uniqueness of Pellet Smoker and Grills lies in the combination of the flavor and versatility it offers. Accurate, Pellet Smoker and Grills make an explosive mixture of sublime tastes and incredible deliciousness; it is a great Smoker and Grill appliance that you can use if you want to enjoy the taste of charcoal grill and at the same time you don't want to give up on the traditional taste of ovens. And what is more interesting about pellet Smoker and Grills is that, with a single button, you can grill, roast, bake, braise and smoke, your favorite meat portions. And things can still get better as pellet Smoker and Grills are automatic, so you can just set the temperature of pellet Smoker and Grill and walk away; then when you are back, you will be able to enjoy great flavors you are craving for. But how can we use a Pellet Smoker and Grill?

How to Use a Wood Pellet Smoker and Grill?

Pellet Smoker and Grills function based on an advanced digital technology and many mechanical parts. The pellet Smoker and Grill are then lit while the temperature is usually programmed with the help of a digital control board. Pellet Smoker and Grills work by using algorithm so that it allows calculating the exact number of pellets you should use in order to reach the perfect temperature. Every Wood Pellet Grill is equipped with a rotating auger that allows to automatically feed the fire right from the hopper to the fire in order to maintain the same temperature. And even as the food continues cooking, the wood pellet Smoker and Grill will continue to drop the exact amount of pellets needed to keep the perfect cooking temperature. But what can we cook with a pellet Smoker and Grill.

What Dishes Can We Can On A Wood Pellet Smoker And Grill?

Thanks to its versatile properties to smoke, grill, braise and kitchen oven, Wood Pellet Smoker and Grill can be used to cook endless dishes and recipes. In fact, there is no actual limit of the recipes you can cook like hot dogs, chicken, vegetables, seafood, rabbit, chicken, brisket, turkey and even more. The cooking process is very easy; all you have to do is to pack your favorite wood pellets into the hopper; then program the temperature you desire on the controller; then place the food on the pellet Smoker and Grill. That is it and the pellet will be able to maintain the temperature and keep the pellets burning.

Pellet Smoker and Grills are characterized by being electric and it requires a usual standard outlet of about 110v so that you can power the digital board, fan and auger.

There is a wide variety of types of pellet smoker and grills, like electric pellet smokers, wood fired grills, wood pellet grills and wood pellet smokers; to name a few pellet Smoker and Grill names. But all these names refer to the same outdoor cooker appliance that is only fueled by hardwood pellets. And there are many brands of Wood Pellet Smoker and Grills, like Traeger.

For instance, Traeger is known for being one of the world's most well-known brands of pellet grills. Indeed, Joe Traeger was the person who invented the pellet grill during the mid-1980s and he gave his name to this invention. And when the Traeger patent expired, many other Pellet Smoker and Grills came to life into the market.

Advantages of Wood Pellet Smoker and Grill

Roasting and grilling meat make two cooking methods that play an important role in packing meat with flavorful tastes. And not only grilling makes a healthier cooking technique, but it can also help retain nutrients within the meat portions. And there is no better and useful machine more than the wood pellet Smoker and Grill that you can use to replace the traditional grilling machine known as barbecue. Indeed, Wood Pellet Smoker and Grill have too many advantages. And here are some of the most well-known benefits of using a Pellet Smoker and Grill:

1. Wood Pellet Smoker and Grills are designed to enhance more flavors and aromas by using as fuel only wood pellets. And by following this method, we can enjoy flavors that we love with a very few ingredients and hardwood pellets.

2. Useful and versatile. Using a wood pellet Smoker and Grill can help you cook a wide variety of dishes and one of the most well-known advantages of this cooking appliance is its versatility. Indeed, wood pellet Smoker

and Grills allow cooking different types of ingredients from braised short ribs to chicken drumsticks and wings.

3. Fast and convenient. Have you ever wanted to find a convenient, fast and effortless cooking appliance or technique that can save your time and effort? Indeed, the pellet Smoker and Grill makes a great choice when it comes to saving time and it deserves to give it a try. The idea behind using a wood pellet smoker cooker stems from its great popularity and pellet Smoker and Grills are quickly preheated; thus it can save you so much time.

4. Pellet Smoker and Grill and Temperature regulation. Using a Pellet Smoker and Grill allows you to monitor the temperature of the inner chamber better by regulating it. And while it is very difficult to manage the level of temperature with traditional smokers and grills; pellet Smoker and Grill makes this mission easier. And pellet Smoker and Grills will help keep the temperature under constant check and to retain the delicious flavors of various ingredients.

5. Variety of pellets. Cooking experts with wooden Pellet Smoker and Grills have studied this cooking appliance very well and they even suggest using your favorite flavors. For instance, pellets exist in different flavors like maple, pecan and hickory wood.

6. Evenly-cooked ingredients. Wood Pellet Smoker and Grills offer a better way to get your food ingredients perfectly cooked from the outside to the inside alike. This appliance uses electricity to function and offers fast and even cooking without any difficulties. Besides, wood pellet Smoker and Grills are equipped with a heat diffuser plate that makes the cooking process easier.

7. Easy to clean. Wood pellet Smoker and Grills are equipped with a catch plate that is placed right under the machine and the function of this plate is to catch the drips during the cooking process. Thus, it becomes very easy to clean the wood pellet Smoker and Grill.

TEMPERATURE CONTROL

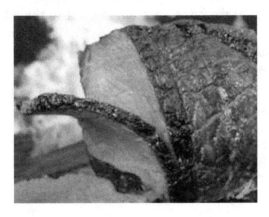

A pellet flame broil is a kind of barbecue that depends on tube-shaped hardwood sawdust pellets as fuel for the barbecuing. The sawdust is sourced from spots, for example, saw factories and timber yard. The wood pellet resembles a long pill and has a breadth of about ¼ inch. The small size of the pellets empowers them to consume neatly without leaving a great deal of fiery debris. A concoction called lignin will be discharged into the smoke when the wood pellets are copied and add a wood terminated flavor to the meat. Other than that, it doesn't contain some other added substance.

What are the Portions of a Pellet Grill?

The enlistment fan guarantees that the smoke from the hardwood pellet is coursed appropriately in the cook chamber. This ensures the flavor is circulated equally on the meat. The twist drill moves the wood pellets into the flame pot. The twist drill can move delayed for low-temperature cooking, or it can run at a quick rate for high-temperature baking.

The warmth diffuser transmits and scatters the warmth equitably on the cooking surface of the barbecue to guarantee that all zones of the meat are cooked well. The dribble dish is situated over the warmth diffuser, and it gets the oil that tumbles from the flame broil. The capacity container is the place you store the wood pellet energies. Topping the capacity container off to the edge keeps you from always having to return to refill it. The speedster will sparkle red and consume the pellets in smoke while you go to unwind and doing different things.

Points of Interest

You can cook practically any sort of meat on the pellet barbecue.

The flame broil can be preheated inside a period of 10 - 15 minutes.

You can set physically set the temperature on the advanced controller anyplace in the middle of 175° F to 500° F. Some pellet flame broils enables you to change the temperature by a 5 ° F increase.

Many pellet barbecues offer Bluetooth include that enables you to utilize a Bluetooth gadget to screen the cooking. It additionally accompanies a meat test for checking the cooking time.

Different sizes of pellet flame broils are accessible from family to business size units. The drunker the capacities, the more costly it is. The business size unit offers more spaces to flame broil meat as enormous overall hoard for a horde of individuals. A portion of the leading brand names is Traeger, Yoder Smokers and Memphis Wood Fire Grills.

The wood pellets that fuel the barbecuing is accessible in a wide range of sorts of flavors including cherry, birch, apple, maple, whiskey and hickory. You can blend the pellets add more than one characters to the meat.

A single 20-pound sack of pellets is adequate for flame broiling the sustenance a few times. The flame broil will expend around 2 pounds of pellets consistently. Be that as it may, the real utilization of the pellets will rely upon different factors, for example, temperature and wind. In case you are fire cooking open air and there happens to be a great deal of wind, you should utilize more pellets to give the fuel.

Burdens

It is subject to power so it might be poorly arranged for you to flame broil the meat in a spot that doesn't have any electrical outlet close by. You have to connect it to a standard 110v electrical outlet in the house.

A pellet barbecue can be costly, and the littlest family unit will cost at any rate a couple of hundred dollars.

There will, in general, be secondary smoke when you set a higher temperature. The best temperature to cook is 250 degrees.

Extra Tips

It is savvy to contribute more cash forthright to purchase a quality pellet flame broil that will keep going for a long time. Pellet flame broils produced using 304 or 430 evaluation tempered steel is the best as they are safe against rust. To see whether a barbecue is a high quality, you can check whether it has an active development including equipment, joints and flame broil. Perusing surveys and posing inquiries on the discussion can assist you with making the correct choice.

1.4 History of Wood Pellet Smoker-Grills

Today there is a multitude of wood pellet smoker-grill manufacturers providing a wide range of excellent barbecue pits. These units cover a broad spectrum, from entry level to sophisticated pits priced from $300 to over $2,500. Just a few decades ago, this was not the case. Wood pellet smoker-grills were first introduced in the 1990s by a small company in Oregon called Traeger Grills. Years ago, I remember watching Traeger commercials featuring Terry Bradshaw, and ogling Traeger grills at my local Ace Hardware store. Those commercials made it look so simply, and I can now attest to the fact that they were right! The industry only grew by leaps and bounds once Traeger's original patent expired. More and more people became exposed to the fabulous, mouth-watering food from a wood pellet smoker-grill, but as recently as 2008 only two companies manufactured wood pellet smoker-grills: Traeger and its rival MAK, also based in Oregon. Today there are more than 20 brands of excellent wood pellet smoker-grill manufacturers carried by a wide range of outlets from local barbecue stores, butcher shops, feed stores, hardware stores, big box stores, online outlets, and direct from the manufacturer.

T he Wood Pellet Grill is not only limited to, well, grilling. It is an essential outdoor kitchen appliance as it allows you also to bake, roast, and smoke, braise, and barbecue. But more than it is a useful kitchen appliance, below are the advantages of getting your very own Wood Pellet Grill:

Better flavor: The Wood Pellet Grill uses all-natural wood, so food comes out better-tasting compared to when you cook them in a gas or charcoal grill.

No flare-ups: No flare-ups mean that food is cooked evenly on all sides. This is made possible by using indirect heat. And because there are no flare-ups, you can smoke, bake, and rise without some areas or sides of your food burning.

Mechanical parts are well designed and protected: The mechanical parts of the Wood Pellet Grill are protected particularly from fats and drippings, so it does not get stuck over time.

Exceptional temperature control: The Wood Pellet Grill has exceptional temperature control. The thing is that all you need is to set up the heat and the grill will maintain a consistent temperature even if the weather goes bad. Moreover, having a stable temperature control allows you to cook food better and tastier minus the burnt taste.

Environmentally friendly: Perhaps the main selling point of the Wood Pellet Grill is that it is environmentally friendly. Wood Pellet Grill uses all-natural wood pellets, so your grill does not produce harmful chemicals when you are using it... only smoky goodness.

The thing is that the Wood Pellet Grill is more than just your average grill. It is one of the best there is, and you will get your money's worth with this grill.

Benefits

To help you enjoy the best of cooking experience and ensure that you truly bring out the best in the recipes, we are going to talk about some of the best tips and tricks that you can make use of.

However, just before that, we want to familiarize you with the key benefits which the use of wood pellet grills has to offer. Make sure to optimize the most out of it.

· **Ease of use: Compared to smokers and even other cooking methods, there is no denying the fact that wood pellet grills offer remarkable ease of use. You can simply feed in the controls and relax and enjoy the meals.**
· **Versatile: The use of wood pellet grills will ensure that you will be able to cook a wide variety of food. There is going to be a massive variety as these grills aren't limited to meat alone. From braised short ribs to poultry, beef, and red meat, chicken, and more; there are a whole lot of things you can work on.**
· **Even cooking: There is no doubt that these grills let you have a very even style of cooking. This, in turn, makes sure that the quality of food is top-notch.**
· **Regulating the temperature: With wood pellet grills, you don't need to babysit the whole time. When it comes to regulating the temperature, the controller will take care of it. With the traditional grills, this is often the most tedious task in the cooking process.**

Different Types for Different Meat Flavors

Types of Smoker Woods

Smoker wood is an important element which you need to decide correctly to cook a delicious smoked food. The reason is that smoker chips of woods impart different flavors on the food you are cooking in the smoker. Therefore, you should know which smoker wood should be used to create a delicious smoked food. Here is the lowdown of smoker woods and which food is best with them.

1- Alder: A lighter smoker wood with natural sweetness.

Best to smoke: Any fish especially salmon, poultry and game birds.

2- Maple: This smoker wood has a mild and sweet flavor. In addition, its sweet smoke gives the food a dark appearance. For better flavor, use it as a combination with alder, apple or oak smoker woods.

Best to smoke: Vegetables, cheese, and poultry.

3- Apple: A mild fruity flavor smoker wood with natural sweetness. When mixed with oak smoker wood, it gives a great flavor to food. Let food smoke for several hours as the smoke takes a while to permeate the food with the flavors.

Best to smoke: Poultry, beef, pork, lamb, and seafood.

4- Cherry: This smoker wood is an all-purpose fruity flavor wood for any type of meat. Its smoke gives the food a rich, mahogany color. Try smoking by mixing it with alder, oak, pecan and hickory smoker wood.

Best to smoke: Chicken, turkey, ham, pork, and beef.

5- Oak: Oakwood gives a medium flavor to food which is stronger compared to apple wood and cherry wood and lighter compared to hickory. This versatile smoker wood works well blended with hickory, apple, and cherry woods.

Best to smoke: Sausages, brisket, and lamb.

6- Peach and Pear: Both smoker woods are similar to each other. They give food a subtle light and fruity flavor with the addition of natural sweetness.

Best to smoke: Poultry, pork and game birds.

7- Hickory: Hickory wood infuses a strong sweet and bacon flavor into the food, especially meat cuts. Don't over smoke with this wood as it can turn the taste of food bitter.

Best to smoke: Red meat, poultry, pork shoulder, ribs.

8- Pecan: This sweet smoker wood lends the food a rich and nutty flavor. Use it with Mesquite wood to balance its sweetness.

Best to smoke: Poultry, pork.

9- Walnut: This strong flavored smoker wood is often used as a mixing wood due to its slightly bitter flavor. Use walnut wood with lighter smoke woods like pecan wood or apple wood.

Best to smoke: Red meat and game birds.

10. Grape: Grape wood chips give a sweet berry flavor to food. It's best to use these wood chips with apple wood chips.

Best to smoke: Poultry

11. Mulberry: Mulberry wood chips are similar to apple wood chips. It adds natural sweetness and gives berry finish to the food.

Best to smoke: Ham and Chicken.

12. Mesquite: Mesquite wood chips flavor is earthy and slightly harsh and bitter. It burns fast and strongly hot. Therefore, don't use it for longer grilling.
Best to smoke: Red meat, dark meat.

Fundamentals Of Wood Pellet Cooking

With the hundreds of different varieties and brands of wood pellets, it is often difficult to identify which brand to consider. If you are not sure what brand to opt for, it might help to try at least the top three brands you know of and compare their efficiency.

Appearance

The first factor to consider when choosing a brand of wood pellets is the appearance of the pellets. After using wood pellets for some time, you will be able to tell and judge their quality simply by how they appear. The first thing to check is the length of the pellets. Brands adhere to certain standards, so this is not a concern. Nevertheless, you need to understand that when it comes to pellet fuels, length matters, as it will affect the performance of the pellets. The dust you will find in the packaging is also another to consider. It is normal to see fines once you open the bag, but if there are an unusual number of fines, it means the pellets aren't of good quality.

Texture

The texture of the pellets is another thing. Wood pellets have a certain texture in them. If you feel that the pellets are smooth and shiny, it means they are of good quality. The same is true if the pellets do not have cracks. If the pellets are too rough with unusual racks on the surface, it means the pellets are bad. This is usually a result of incorrect pressing ratio and moisture content of the raw materials used in making the pellets.

Smell

Wood pellets are made by exposing them to high temperatures within a sealed space. During the process, the lignin contained in the biomass material is mixed with other elements, producing a smell of burnt fresh wood. If the pellets smell bad, there is a huge chance they have not been processed properly or contain impure, raw material.

Aside from the appearance, texture, and smell of the wood pellets, another way to check their quality is to see how they react with water. Place a handful of pellets in a bowl of water and allow them to settle for several minutes. If the pellets dissolve in the water and expand quickly, this means they are of good quality. On the other hand, if the pellets do not dissolve within minutes but instead expand and become hard, it means they are of bad quality.

Finally, try burning some of the pellets, as well. If the wood pellets are of excellent quality, the flame they produce will be bright and brown. If the flame they produce, on the other hand, is dark in color, it means the quality of the pellets is not good. Also, good-quality pellets produce a little ash, so if the pellets leave you with a lot of residues, it is a sign that the pellets are bad.

Right Wood For Right Meat, Right Temperature

Choose the type of meat that tastes good with a smoky flavor. Following meat goes well for smoking.

Beef: ribs, brisket, and corned beef.

Pork: spareribs, roast, shoulder, and ham.

Poultry: whole chicken, a whole turkey, and big game hens.

Seafood: Salmon, scallops, trout, and lobster.

With so many recipes to try with your pellet grill, it is easy to get overwhelmed right away. One important thing to keep in mind is that lower temperatures produce smoke, while higher temperatures do not. Follow this useful guide below to know the temperature and time it requires to get the perfectly flavored meat each time.

· **Beef briskets are best cooked at 250 degrees using the smoke setting for at least 4 hours by itself and covered with foil for another 4 hours.**
· **Pork ribs should be cooked at 275 degrees on the smoke setting for 3 hours and covered with foil for another 2-3 hours.**
· **Steaks require 400-450 degrees for about 10 minutes each side.**
· **Turkey can be cooked at 375 degrees for 20 minutes per pound of meat. For smoked turkey, the heat settings should be around 180-225 degrees for 10-12 hours or until the inside of the turkey reaches 165 degrees.**
· **Chicken breasts can be cooked at 400-450 degrees for 15 minutes on each side.**
· **A whole chicken cooks at 400-450 degrees for 1.5 hours or until the internal temperature reaches 165 degrees.**
· **Bacon and sausage can be cooked at 425 degrees for 5-8 minutes on each side.**
· **Hamburgers should be cooked at 350 degrees for at least 8 minutes for each side.**
· **You can smoke salmon for 1-1.5 hours and finish with a high setting for 2-3 minutes on each side.**
· **Shrimps cook at 400-450 degrees for 3-5 minutes on each side. If you prefer a smokier flavor, set the temperature at 225 degrees for about 30 minutes.**

Difference Between Hot And Cold Smoking

Cold smoking

Usually, the Smokehouse temperature for cold smoking is around 68-86 degrees F. In this process, the food is not cooked or smoked, cold smoking only provides a Smokey flavor to it, and still, the meat and vegetables remain moist. This technique is mostly a flavor enhancer for the food, which is, later, going to be roasted, baked, or cooked in any other process rather than smoking.

To cold-smoke meat like a pro, you will need to measure preservatives and salt correctly, set the temperature of the smoker rightly, measure the internal temperature of the meat with a high-quality thermometer, clean and maintain the chamber of the smoker properly and finally safely store meat to avoid bacteria growth (sodium nitrate can help to prevent bacteria growth).

Hot smoking

In hot smoking, we use a combination of heat and smoke to cook food and get them served immediately. Most food cooked by this method is marinated for hours before being cooked. Hence, there is no need for curing since the meat/food is prepared and served immediately.

Hot Smoking occurs between the temperatures of 126-176 degrees F. In this temperature, the food is thoroughly cooked, moist, and very flavorful. In hot smoking, it is not preferred to smoke the food in more than 186 degrees F because doing so will make the food shrink excessively, lose all its moisture and fat content, and reduces the yield. The time required for smoking varies depending on the type of food that is being hot smoked. When carrying out hot smoking, there is a need to pay attention to the internal temperature of the food.

Basic Preparations

Getting Meat Ready

Prepare meat according to the recipe. Sometimes meat is cured, marinated, or simply seasoned with the rub. These preparation methods ensure smoked meat turns out flavorful, tender, and extremely juicy.

Brine is a solution to treating poultry, pork, or ham. It involves dissolving brine ingredients in water poured into a huge container and then adding meat to it. Then let soak for at least 8 hours and after that, rinse it well and pat dry before you begin smoking.

Marinate treat beef or briskets and add flavors to it. It's better to make deep cuts in meat to let marinate ingredients deep into it. Drain meat or smoke it straightaway.

Rubs are commonly used to treat beef, poultry, or ribs. They are a combination of salt and many spices, rubbed generously all over the meat. Then the meat is left to rest for at least 2 hours or more before smoking it.

Before smoking meat, make sure it is at room temperature. This ensures the meat is cooked evenly and reaches its internal temperature at the end of the smoking time.

Grilling Tips

So, now let us focus on some of the best tips and tricks you can use to become a smart chef and ace the art of using the wood pellet grill.

- Never ignore the use of upper racks. If you can place a water pan beneath the rack, it will allow for even better cooking.
- Always make it a point to choose the right pellets when using the grill. If you want to have a specific flavor, use flavored wood pellets. You also have mixed variants. Mostly, the food-grade version is a recommended choice.
- When the 40-pound bag of pellet is gone, make sure to clean the grill thoroughly. This will add to the longevity of your grill.
- You should make it a point to soak the wood chips in water before you start cooking. This greatly enhances the flavor.

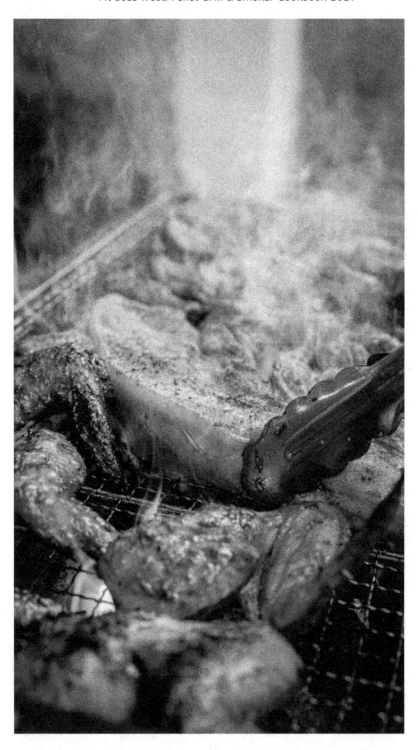

Appetizers And Sides Recipes

1. Bacon Cheddar Slider

Preparation Time: 30 Minutes

Cooking Time: 15 Minutes

Servings: 6 To 10

Ingredients:

- 1 pound ground beef (80% lean)

- ½ teaspoon of garlic salt

- ½ teaspoon salt

- ½ teaspoon of garlic

- ½ teaspoon onion

- ½ teaspoon black pepper

- 6 bacon slices, cut in half

- ½ Cup mayonnaise

- 2 teaspoons of creamy wasabi (optional)

- 6 sliced sharp cheddar cheese, cut in half (optional)

- Sliced red onion

- ½ Cup sliced kosher dill pickles

- 12 mini breads sliced horizontally

- Ketchup

Directions:

1. Place ground beef, garlic salt, seasoned salt, garlic powder, onion powder and black hupe pepper in a medium bowl.

2. Divide in 12 equal parts the meat mixture into shape into small thin round patties (about 2 ounces each) and save.

3. Cook the bacon on medium heat over medium heat for 5-8 minutes until crunchy. Set aside.

4. To make the sauce, mix the mayonnaise and horseradish in a small bowl, if used.

5. Set up a wood pellet smoker and grill for direct cooking to use griddle accessories. Look for the manufacturer

to see if there is a griddle accessory that works with the particular wooden pellet smoker and grill.

6. Spray a cooking spray on the griddle cooking surface for best non-stick results.

7. Preheat wood pellet smoker and grill to 350 ° F using selected pellets. Griddle surface should be approximately 400 ° F.

8. Grill the putty for 3-4 minutes each until the internal temperature reaches 160 ° F.

9. If necessary, place a sharp cheddar cheese slice on each patty while the patty is on the griddle or after the patty is removed from the griddle. Place a small amount of mayonnaise mixture, a slice of red onion, and a hamburger pate in the lower half of each roll. Pickled slices, bacon and ketchup

Nutrition: Calories: 80 Carbs: 0g Fat: 5g Protein: 0g

2. Apple Wood Smoked Cheese

Preparation Time: 1 Hour 15 Minutes

Cooking Time: 2 Hours

Servings: 6

Ingredients:

- Gouda

- Sharp cheddar

- Very sharp 3 year cheddar

- Monterey Jack

- Pepper jack

- Swiss

Directions:

1. According to the shape of the cheese block, cut the cheese block into an easy-to-handle size (approximately 4 x 4 inch block) to promote smoke penetration.

2. Leave the cheese on the counter for one hour to form a very thin skin or crust, which acts as a heat barrier, but allows smoke to penetrate.

3. Configure the wood pellet smoking grill for indirect heating and install a cold smoke box to prepare for cold smoke. Make sure that the louvers on the smoking box are fully open to allow moisture to escape from the box.

4. Preheat the wood pellet smoker and grill to 180 ° F or use apple pellets and smoke settings, if any, to get a milder smoke flavor.

5. Place the cheese on a Teflon-coated fiberglass non-stick grill mat and let cool for 2 hours.

6. Remove the smoked cheese and cool for 1 hour on the counter using a cooling rack.

7. After labelling the smoked cheese with a vacuum seal, refrigerate for 2 weeks or more, then smoke will permeate and the cheese flavor will become milder.

Nutrition: Calories: 102 Carbs: 0g Fat: 9g Protein: 6g

3. Hickory Smoked Moink Ball Skewer

Preparation Time: 30 Minutes

Cooking Time: 1 Hour 30 Minutes

Servings: 9

Ingredients:

- ½ pound ground beef (80% lean)

- ½ pound pork sausage

- 1 large egg

- ½ cup Italian bread crumbs

- ½ cup chopped red onion

- Grated parmesan cheese cup

- ¼ Cup finely chopped parsley

- ¼ cup whole milk

- 2 pieces of garlic, 1 chopped or crushed garlic

- 1 teaspoon oregano

- ½ teaspoon kosher salt

- ½ teaspoon black pepper

- ¼ cup barbecue sauce like Sweet Baby Ray

- ½ pound bacon cut in half, cut in half

Directions:

1. In a container, mix ground beef, ground pork sausage, eggs, crumbs, onions, parmesan cheese, parsley, milk, garlic, salt, oregano, and pepper. Do not overuse the meat.

2. Form a 1½ ounces meatball about 1.5 inches in diameter and place on a Teflon-coated fiberglass mat.

3. Wrap each meatball in half thin bacon. Stab moink balls on 6 skewers (3 balls per skewer).

4. Set up wood pellet smoker and grill for indirect cooking.

5. Preheat wood pellet smoker and grill to 225 ° F using hickory pellets.

6. Tap the moink ball skewer for 30 minutes.

7. Raise the pit temperature to 350 ˚ F until the meatball internal temperature reaches 175 ˚ F and the bacon is crisp (about 40-45 minutes).

8. For the last 5 minutes, brush your moink ball with your favorite barbecue sauce.

9. While still hot, offer moink ball skewers.

Nutrition: Calories: 170 Carbs: 2g Fat: 15g Protein: 7g

Beef Recipes

4. Italian Beef Sandwich

Ingredients:

- 1 Qty. (4 Lb.) Lean, Boneless Beef Roast (Sirloin or Top Round)

- Salt

- Pepper

- 4 Cloves Garlic, Thinly Sliced

- Traeger Prime Rib Rub

- 6 Cups Beef Broth 8 Hoagie-Style Buns (For Sandwiches)

- 6 Slices Swiss Cheese

- 1 Cup Bottled Giardiniera (Italian Pickled Vegetables; Optional), Chopped

Instructions:

- When ready to cook, set the temperature to 450°F and preheat, lid closed for 15 minutes.

- Season the roast liberally with salt, pepper and Traeger prime rib rub. Using a paring knife, make 10-15 slits in the roast every 1" or so. Insert a garlic clove into each slit.

- Place the roast directly on the grill grate and cook for about 1 hour flipping halfway through until browned well.

- Remove the roast from the grill and transfer to a deep Dutch oven. Pour the beef broth over the roast. Cover tightly with foil and place back on the grill. Reduce the grill temperature to 300°F and cook the roast for 3-4 hours or until it is fork tender.

- While the roast cooks, chop the giardiniera into small pieces.

- Remove the Dutch oven from the grill and shred removing any large bits of fat or connective tissue. Transfer the meat back to the Dutch over and stir to combine with the juices.

- Increase the grill temperature to high and preheat lid closed for 10 minutes.

- Place hoagie buns cut side up on a small sheet tray. Fill with the shredded roast and top with a slice of cheese.

Transfer to the grill and cook for another 5-10 minutes or until the cheese is melted.

- Remove from the grill and top with chopped pickled veggies. Serve with remaining cooking liquid for dipping if desired. Enjoy!

5. Thai Beef Skewers

Ingredients:

- 1/4 Cup Vegetable Oil

- 1/4 Cup Soy Sauce

- 1 Juice of Lime

- 2 Cloves Garlic, Finely Minced

- 1 Tbsp. Fresh Ginger, Peeled and Minced

- 1 Tsp. Black Pepper, Freshly Ground

- 1/2 Beef Sirloin, Trimmed and Cut Into 1-1/4 Inch Dice

- 1/2 Red Bell Pepper, Stemmed, Seeded, And Cut Into 1/4 Inch Dice

- 1/2 Cup Dry-Roasted Peanuts (Salted or Unsalted), Coarsely Chopped 1 Traeger Skewers Set

Instructions:

- In a small bowl, whisk together the oil, soy sauce, lime juice, garlic, ginger, sugar, and black pepper. Transfer the meat to a large bowl or resealable plastic bag and pour the marinade over the meat, turning to coat each piece thoroughly. Refrigerate for 2 to 4 hours, or longer if desired.

- Drain the marinade off the sirloin cubes (discard the marinade) and pat them dry with paper towels. Thread the meat on the skewers, keeping the pieces close together to minimize exposure of the skewer to the heat. (You can also slip a folded length of aluminum foil under the exposed ends to protect them.)

- When ready to cook, set the temperature to 425°F and preheat, lid closed for 15 minutes.

- Arrange the skewers on the grill grate and grill for 2 to 4 minutes per side, or until the desired degree of doneness is reached. To serve, sprinkle with the diced red pepper and the chopped peanuts. Enjoy!

6. BBQ CHILI BURGER

Ingredients:

- Beef Chili

- 2.5 Lbs. Ground Beef

- 1 Large Onion, Diced

- 1 Tsp Kosher Salt

- 1 Can Chipotles in Adobo, Minced with Sauce

- 1/4 Cup Chili Powder

- 1-1/2 Tbsp Cumin Powder

- 3 Cloves Garlic, Peeled and Minced

- 1 Jalapeño Pepper, Minced

- 1 (14 Oz) Can Diced or Crushed Tomatoes

- 2 Cups Chicken Stock

- 1/8 Cup Flour

- 1/2 Tbsp Dark Chili Powder

- 1/2 Tbsp Ground Cinnamon

- Juice Of 1 Lime

- 1 Hershey's Chocolate Bar

- Salt and Pepper, To Taste

- Chili Burgers

- 2 Lbs. Ground Beef

- Traeger Beef Rub, As Needed

- 2 Cups Beef Chili or Preferred Chili

- 5 Hamburger Buns

- 5 Slices Cheddar Cheese

- 1 Red Onion, Sliced

- 1 Bag Frito Corn Chips

Instructions:

- For the Beef Chili: Heat a large Dutch oven on the stove top over medium-high heat. Cook the ground beef until browned and cooked through.

- Add all chili Ingredients: minus the chocolate and limes to the Dutch oven.

- When ready to cook, start the Traeger according to grill instructions. Set the temperature to 350 degrees F and preheat, lid closed for 10 to 15 minutes.

- Put the Dutch oven into the grill for 2 hours, stirring every hour. Remove Dutch oven from grill.

- Stir the lime juice and the chocolate into the chili. Set chili aside until ready to assemble the burgers.

- For the burgers: When ready to cook, set the temperature to 350°F and preheat, lid closed for 15 minutes.

- Form into 5 equal patties and season both sides with Traeger Beef Rub.

- Place patties directly on the grill grate and cook for 4-5 minutes per side, flipping once. Top each burger with cheese and cook for 1 minute more to melt.

- Remove from the grill and let rest 1-2 minutes.

- To build burger, place the patty on the bottom bun, add a scoop of chili, Fritos, red onion and finish with the top bun. Enjoy

7. Traeger Filet Mignon

Ingredients:

- 3 Filet Mignon Steaks

- 1 Tsp Salt

- 1 Tsp Pepper

- 2 Cloves Garlic, Minced

- 3 Tbsp Butter, Softened

Instructions:

- In a small bowl combine salt, pepper, garlic, and softened butter. Rub on both sides of filets. Let rest 10 minutes.

- When ready to cook, set the temperature to 450°F and preheat, lid closed for 15 minutes.

- Place steaks directly on the grill and cook for 5-8 minutes on each side, or until the filets reach an internal temperature of 135-140 degrees F for medium rare. Enjoy!

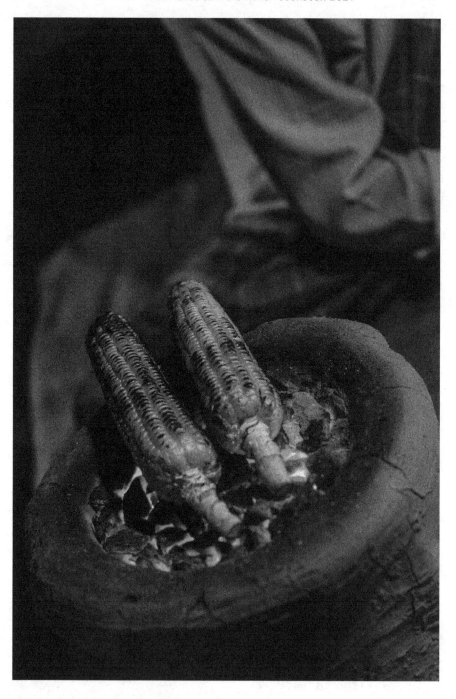

Lamp Recipes

8. Grilled Lamb Burgers with Pickled Onions

Ingredients:

- Pickled Onions

- 1/2 Red Onion, Thinly Sliced

- 6 Tbsp Lime Juice

- 1/2 Tsp Kosher Salt

- 1/2 Tsp Raw Cane Sugar

- Yogurt Sauce

- 1 Cup Greek Yogurt

- 2 Tbsp Lemon Juice

- 1 Garlic Clove, Minced

- 2 Tbsp Finely Chopped Herbs, Such as Mint, Dill and Parsley

- 1/2 Tsp Kosher Salt

- Lamb Burgers

- 1 Tbsp Olive Oil

- 1/2 Red Onion, Finely Diced

- 1 Lb. Ground Lamb

- 8 Oz Ground Pork

- 3 Tbsp Finely Chopped Mint

- 2 Tbsp Finely Chopped Dill

- 3 Tbsp Finely Chopped Parsley

- 4 Garlic Cloves, Minced

- 1 1/2 Tsp Ground Cumin

- 1 Tsp Ground Coriander

- 1 Tsp Kosher Salt

- 1/2 Tsp Freshly Ground Black Pepper

- 1 Sliced Tomato

- 6 Buns

- Sliced Cucumber

- Butter Lettuce

Instructions:

- To Pickle the Onions: Place the onion, lime juice, salt and sugar in a small bowl. Stir to combine, cover and let sit at room temperature for about 2 hours to soften. Refrigerate until ready to use.

- To make the Yogurt Sauce: In a small bowl, stir together the yogurt, lemon juice, garlic, herbs, and 1/2 tsp salt. Adjust the salt to taste. Cover and refrigerate until ready to serve, or for up to 2 days.

- To make the lamb burgers: In a small skillet over medium heat, warm the olive oil. Add the onion and cook, stirring frequently until softened, about 7 minutes. Transfer to a small plate to cool.

- In a large bowl, combine the lamb, pork, mint, dill, parsley, garlic, cumin, coriander, salt, pepper, and cooled onions. Gently mix with your hands. Do not overwork the meat.

- Divide the mixture into 6 equal balls. Press into patties and transfer to a parchment-lined baking sheet. If not cooking immediately, cover and refrigerate for up to 8 hours.

- When ready to cook, set the temperature to High and preheat, lid closed for 15 minutes.

- Place the burgers on the grill and cook until well-browned, about 2 to 3 minutes per side for medium-rare, or about 5 minutes per side for well done.

- Transfer burgers to a plate to rest for 5 minutes before serving.

- Place burgers on buns and top with a generous dollop of herbed yogurt sauce and some pickled onions.

- Add lettuce, sliced tomatoes or cucumbers if desired. Serve immediately. Enjoy!

9. Braised Lamb Shank

Ingredients:

- 4 Shanks Lamb

- Olive Oil, As Needed

- Traeger Prime Rib Rub

- 1 Cup Beef Broth

- 1 Cup Red Wine

- 4 Sprigs Fresh Rosemary and Thyme

Instructions:

- Season the lamb shanks liberally with Traeger Prime Rib Rub.

- When ready to cook, set the temperature to High and preheat, lid closed for 15 minutes.

- Place the shanks directly on the grill grate and cook for 20 minutes or until the exterior has browned.

- Transfer the shanks to a Dutch oven and pour in beef broth, wine, and add herbs. Cover with a tight-fitting lid and place back on the grill grate reducing the temperature to 325°F .

- Braise the shanks for 3-4 hours until the internal temperature is 180°F . Take care not to touch bone with the tip of the temperature probe or you will get a false reading.

- Carefully lift the lid and transfer the lamb and any accumulated juices to a platter or plates. Enjoy!

10. Greek Style Roast Leg of Lamb Recipe

Ingredients:

- One 6-7 Lbs. Leg of Lamb, Bone-In

- 8 Cloves Garlic

- 2 Sprigs Fresh Rosemary, Needles Stripped, Stems Discarded

- 1 Sprig (Or 1 Tsp. Dried) Fresh Oregano

- 2 Lemons, Juiced

- 6 Tbsp. Evo (Extra-Virgin Olive Oil)

- As Needed Coarse Salt (Kosher) And Black Pepper, Freshly Ground

Instructions:

- Using a paring knife, make a series of small slits in the leg.

- On a cutting board, finely mince the garlic, rosemary, and oregano with a chef's knife to make an herb and garlic paste. (Alternatively, put the garlic and herbs in a small food processor.)

- Stuff a small amount of the paste into each of the slits, driving it into the slit with a spoon handle or other utensil. Put the lamb on a rack inside a roasting pan. If desired, like the pan with foil for easier clean-up.
- Rub the outside of the lamb with the lemon juice, then the olive oil. Cover with plastic wrap and refrigerate for at least 8 hours, or overnight.
- Remove from the refrigerator and let the lamb come to room temperature.
- Remove the plastic wrap and season the lamb with salt and pepper. When ready to cook, start the Traeger grill on Smoke with the lid open until the fire is established (4 to 5 minutes). Set the temperature to 400F and preheat, lid closed, for 10 to 15 minutes.
- Roast the lamb for 30 minutes. Reduce the heat to 350F (300 if you have a manual controller) and continue to cook until the internal temperature in the thickest part of the meat - be sure the temperature probe is not touching bone - is about 140F for medium-

rare, about 1 hour more, longer if you're cooking at 300F or prefer your lamb more well-done.

- Transfer the lamb to a cutting board and let rest for 15 minutes before slicing on a diagonal into thin slices.

222

11. Smoked Lamb Sausage

Ingredients:

- Smoked Lamb Sausage
- 2 Lb. Lamb Shoulder
- 1 Qty. (60 Inch) Hog Casing
- 1 Tbsp. Garlic
- 1 Tsp. Cumin
- 1 Tsp. Paprika
- 1/2 Tsp. Cayenne
- 2 Tbsp. Ground Fennel
- 1 Tbsp. Cilantro, Finely Chopped
- 1 Tbsp. Parsley, Finely Chopped
- 1 Tsp. Black Pepper
- 2 Tbsp. Salt
- Sauce

- 3 Cups Greek Yogurt

- 1 Lemon, Juiced

- 1 Clove Garlic

- 1 Cucumber, Peeled, Shredded, And Drained

- 1 Tbsp. Dill

- To Taste Salt & Pepper

Instructions:

- Cut the lamb shoulder into 2-inch pieces, and using a meat grinder, grind the meat.

- Lightly combine the lamb with all the spices in a bowl and refrigerate. It is important to refrigerate the ground lamb so the fat does not melt in order to give the sausage a good texture.

- Next, using a sausage horn, attach the hog casing and start to feed the sausage back through the grinder to fill the casing and twist into links. With a paring knife, prick holes all along the casing (this will allow steam to escape while cooking). Refrigerate. Combine all

- When ready to cook, start your Traeger on Smoke, with the lid open until the fire is established (4 to 5 minutes). Set the temperature to 225°F, place the prepared sausage on the grill grate and smoke it for 1 hour.

- Once the hour is up, remove the links from the grill and turn the grill up to High (450°F) and preheat (10-15 minutes). Once the grill has reached 450°F, place the links back on the grill and cook for 5 minutes on each side.

- Serve hot with yogurt sauce and roasted potatoes on the side. Enjoy!

12. Lamb Lollipops with Mango Chutney

Ingredients:

- Lamb Lollipops

- 6 Lamb Chops, Around 3/4-Inch-Thick, Frenched

- 2 Tbsp Olive Oil

- 1/2 Tsp Course Kosher Salt

- 1/2 Tsp Black Pepper, Freshly Cracked

- 2 Tbsp Fresh Mint, Chopped

- Mango Chutney

- 1 Mango, Peeled, Seeded and Chopped

- 3 Cloves Garlic, Chopped

- 1/2 Habanero Pepper, Seeded and Chopped, Or More to Taste

- 3 Sprigs Fresh Cilantro, Chopped

- 1 Tbsp Fresh Lime Juice

- 1 Teaspoon Salt

- 1/2 Tsp Pepper, Freshly Cracked

Instructions:

- If you can't purchase frenched lamb chops, using a sharp knife, cut and scrape the flesh and fat off the bone to make it look like a lollipop.

- Add all chutney Ingredients into a food processor and pulse about 15 times or until desired consistency; set aside. Chop mint and set aside.

- When ready to cook, start the Traeger grill on Smoke with the lid open until the fire is established (4 to 5 minutes). Set the temperature to High and preheat, lid closed, for 10 to 15 minutes.

- While grill preheats, on a baking sheet drizzle lamb lollipop with olive. Coat both sides. Season both sides with salt and pepper and allow to sit at room temperature for 5 to 10 minutes.

- Place the lamb pops directly on grill grate. Close lid and grill for 5 minutes. Flip over and grill for another 3 minutes or until a thermometer inserted into the thickest part of the meat registers an internal temperature of 130 degrees F.

- Remove from grill and allow to rest 10 minutes before serving.

- Spoon chutney over each lamb lollipop and sprinkle with fresh chopped mint. Enjoy!

13.   Grilled Lamb Chops

Preparation Time: 1 Hour

Cooking Time: 8 Minutes

Servings: 3

Ingredients

- 2 garlic cloves, crushed

- 1 tablespoons rosemary leaves, fresh chopped

- 2 tablespoons olive oil

- 1 tablespoon lemon juice, fresh

- 1 tablespoon thyme leaves, fresh

- 1 tablespoon salt

- 9 lamb loin chops

Directions:

1. Add the garlic, rosemary, oil, juice, salt, and thyme in a food processor. Pulse until smooth.

2. Rub the marinade on the lamb chops both sides and let marinate for 1 hour in a fridge. Tke it from the fridge

and let sit at room temperature for 20 minutes before cooking.

3. Preheat your wood pellet smoker to high heat. Smoke the lamb chops for 5 minutes on each side.

4. Sear the lamb chops for 3 minutes on each side. Remove from the grill and serve with a green salad.

Nutrition: Calories 1140 Fat 99g Carbs 1g Protein 55g

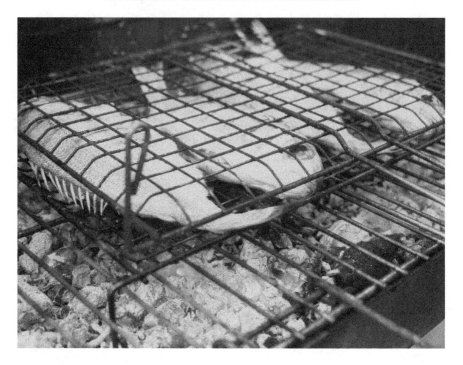

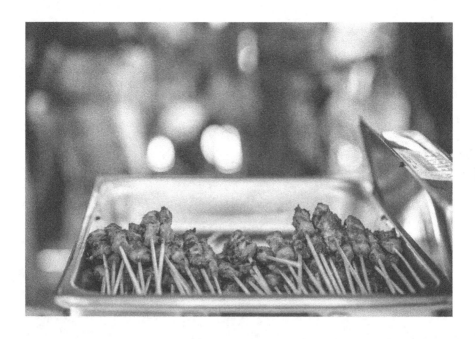

Chicken Recipes

14.   Spicy BBQ Chicken

Ingredients:

- 1 Whole Chicken

- 6 Thai Chiles

- 2 Tbsp Sweet Paprika

- 1 Scotch Bonnet

- 2 Tbsp Sugar

- 3 Tbsp Salt

- 1 White Onion

- 5 Garlic Cloves

- 4 Cups Grape Seed Oil

Instructions:

- Puree the Thai chilies, paprika, scotch bonnet, sugar, salt, onion, garlic, and grape seed oil together until smooth.

- Smother the chicken with mixture and let rest in fridge overnight.

- When ready to cook, set the Traeger to 300°F and preheat, lid closed for 15 minutes.

- Place chicken on grill breast side up and smoke for 3 hours or until it reaches an internal temperature of 165°F in the breast.

- Remove from grill and allow to rest for 10 to 15 minutes before slicing.Serve with sides of choice. Enjoy!

15. Traeger BBQ Half Chickens

Ingredients:

- 1 Ea. (3-3 1/2 Lb.) Young Fresh Chicken

- Traeger Apricot BBQ Sauce

- Traeger Summer Shandi Rub

Instructions:

- Place the chicken, breast side down, on a cutting board with the neck pointing away from you. Cut along one side of the backbone, staying as close to the bone as possible, from the neck to the tail.

- Repeat on the other side of the backbone then remove it. Open the chicken and slice through the white cartilage at the tip of the breastbone to pop it open. Cut down either side of the breast bone then use your fingers to pull it out.

- Flip the chicken over so it is skin side up and cut down the center splitting the chicken in half. Tuck the wings back of each chicken half.

- Season on both sides with Traeger Summer Shandi rub.

- When ready to cook, set the temperature to 375°F and preheat, lid closed for 15 minutes.

- Place chicken directly on the grill grate skin side up and cook until the internal temperature reaches 160 degrees F, about 60-90 minutes.

- Brush the BBQ sauce all over the chicken skin and cook for an additional 10 minutes.

- Remove from grill and let rest 5 minutes before serving. Enjoy!

16.   Smoked Deviled Eggs

Ingredients:

- 7 Hard Boiled Eggs, Cooked and Peeled

- 3 Tbsp Mayonnaise

- 3 Tsp Chives, Diced

- 1 Tsp Brown Mustard

- 1 Tsp Apple Cider Vinegar

- Dash of Hot Sauce

- Salt and Pepper, To Taste

- 2 Tbsp Bacon, Crumbled

- Paprika, For Dusting

Instructions:

- When ready to cook, set temperature to 180°F and preheat, lid closed for 15 minutes. For optimal flavor, use Super Smoke if available.

- Place cooked and peeled eggs directly on the grill grate and smoke eggs for 30 minutes. Remove from grill and allow eggs to cool.

- Slice the eggs lengthwise and scoop the egg yolks into a gallon zip top bag. Add mayonnaise, chives, mustard, vinegar, hot sauce, salt, and pepper to the bag.

- Zip the bag closed and, using your hands, knead all of the Ingredients: together until completely smooth.

- Squeeze the yolk mixture into one corner of the bag and cut a small part of the corner off. Pipe the yolk mixture into the hardboiled egg whites.

- Top the deviled eggs with crumbled bacon and paprika. Chill until ready to serve. Enjoy!

17. Pickled Brined Hot Chicken Sandwich

Ingredients:

- Pickle Brined Chicken

- 2 Cups Leftover Pickle Juice

- 8 Ea. Boneless Skinless Chicken Thighs

- Salt and Pepper, As Needed

- 1 Cup Flour

- 1/2 Cup Tapioca Flour

- 1 Cup Buttermilk

- 2 Tsp Franks Red Hot Sauce

- 1 Egg

- Butter Hot Sauce

- 1/2 Cup Butter, Melted

- 1/2 Cup Franks Red Hot Sauce

- 2 Tsp Cayenne

- 1/2 Tsp Dark Brown Sugar

- 1 Tsp Black Pepper

- 1 Tsp Garlic

- 1 Tsp Paprika

- Sandwich

- Shredded Cabbage Slaw

- Traeger Smoked Pickles

- 4 Sesame Seed Buns

Instructions:

- In a medium bowl, combine pickle juice and chicken thighs. Weigh them down if necessary, to make sure they are completely submerged. Place in the refrigerator to brine overnight.

- When ready to cook, set the temperature to High and preheat, lid closed for 15 minutes.

- Place a cast iron pan with 1/2-inch canola oil on the grill grate while the grill preheats.

- Remove the chicken thighs from the pickle brine and pat dry.

- In a medium bowl combine both flours and a pinch of salt. Mix well to combine.

- In another bowl combine the buttermilk, hot sauce, egg and a pinch of salt. Mix well to combine.

- Season the chicken thighs with salt. Dip the thighs in the flour mixture, then buttermilk, then back into the flour mixture. Transfer to a wire rack and repeat with the remaining thighs.

- Place wire rack directly on the grill grate next to the cast iron of oil and bake chicken for 15 minutes or until the internal temperature reaches 150°F .

- As chicken pieces come to temperature, transfer them 2 or 3 at a time to the preheated oil to crisp the coating and finish cooking.

- For the Butter Hot Sauce: While the chicken is cooking, melt the butter and combine with the hot sauce, brown sugar, cayenne, garlic powder, paprika and black pepper in a medium bowl. Set aside.

- Remove chicken from the oil when the internal temperature reaches 165°F and dunk in the butter hot sauce mixture.

- Build the sandwiches with buns, mayonnaise, pickles, cabbage slaw and hot chicken. Enjoy!

18.   Baked Chicken Cordon Bleu

Ingredients:

- 4 Ea. (4-5 Oz) Boneless, Skinless Chicken Breasts

- 8 Slices Prosciutto or Ham

- 8 Slices Swiss Cheese

- 1/3 Cup All-Purpose Flour

- Salt, As Needed

- Freshly Ground Black Pepper, As Needed

- 1 Cup Dry Breadcrumbs, Preferably Panko

- 1/4 Cup Grated Parmesan Cheese

- 2 Tbsp Melted Butter

- 2 Tsp Fresh Thyme Leaves 2 Eggs

Instructions:

- Spray a baking sheet with nonstick cooking spray. Set aside.

- Butterfly each chicken breast and place between two pieces of plastic wrap. Evenly pound with the flat side of a meat mallet, being careful not to tear the chicken, until chicken is 1/4-inch thick.

- Lay each chicken breast on a fresh piece of plastic wrap. Season chicken with salt and lay 1 to 2 slices of cheese on each breast followed by prosciutto or ham, then 1-2 more slices of cheese.

- Roll the chicken breast up like you would roll a burrito. Using the bottom piece of plastic wrap as an aid, fold the bottom of the breast up about an inch, then fold in the sides. Roll tightly.

- Wrap in the plastic wrap and tightly twist the ends to shape and compress the chicken. Repeat with the remaining chicken breasts. Chill in the refrigerator for 60 minutes.

- While chicken chills, season the flour with salt and pepper and put in a shallow dish.

- Combine the breadcrumbs, parmesan cheese, butter, and thyme. Season with salt and pepper and put in a second shallow dish.

- Whisk the eggs in a separate third dish.

- Arrange your workspace in this order: flour, eggs, breadcrumbs. Put the prepared baking sheet next to the breadcrumbs.

- Remove the plastic wrap from the chicken breasts. Coat each lightly with flour then dip in the egg.

- Finally, roll in breadcrumbs, patting them to make them adhere. Arrange on the baking sheet.

- When ready to cook, set the temperature to 375°F and preheat, lid closed for 15 minutes.

- Place the baking sheet with the chicken on the grill. Bake for 30-40 minutes, or until the coating is golden brown and the chicken is cooked through.

- Serve whole or slice crosswise into pinwheels with a sharp serrated knife. Enjoy!

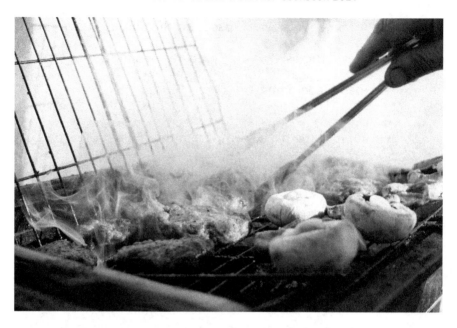

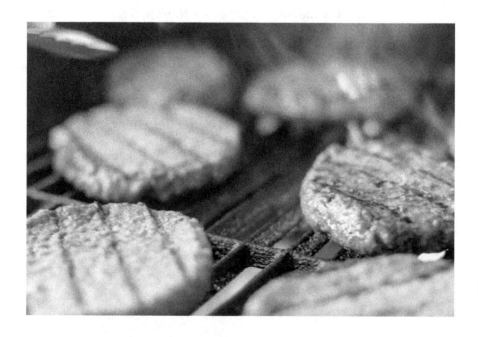

Turkey Recipes

19.   Turkey Jalapeno Meatballs

Ingredients:

- Turkey Jalapeño Meatballs

- 1 1/4 Lbs. Ground Turkey

- 1 Jalapeño Pepper, Deseeded and Finely Diced

- 1/2 Tsp Garlic Salt

- 1 Tsp Onion Powder

- 1 Tsp Salt

- 1/2 Tsp Ground Black Pepper

- 1/4 Tsp Worcestershire Sauce

- Cayenne Pepper, Pinch

- 1 Large Egg, Beaten

- 1/4 Cup Milk

- 1/2 Cup Plain Bread Crumbs Or Panko

- Glaze

- 1 Cup Canned Jellied Cranberry Sauce

- 1/2 Cup Orange Marmalade

- 1/2 Cup Chicken Broth

- 1 Tbsp Jalapeño Pepper, Minced

- Salt, To Taste

- Ground Black Pepper, To Taste

Instructions:

- In a separate small bowl, combine the milk and bread crumbs.

- In a large bowl, mix together turkey, garlic salt, onion powder, salt, pepper, Worcestershire sauce, cayenne pepper, egg and jalapeños.

- Add the bread crumb milk mixture to the bowl and combine. Cover with plastic and refrigerate for up to 1 hour.

- When ready to cook, set the temperature to 350°F and preheat, lid closed for 15 minutes

- Roll the turkey mixture into balls, about one tablespoon each and place the meatballs in a single layer on a parchment lined baking sheet.

- Cook meatballs until they start to brown, flipping occasionally until they reach an internal temperature of 175 degrees F and all sides are browned (about 20 minutes).

- Glaze: Combine cranberry sauce, marmalade, chicken broth, and jalapeños and cook over medium heat in a small saucepan on the stovetop. Cook until Ingredients: are incorporated.

- Half way through meatball cook time, brush the meatballs with the cranberry glaze.

- Transfer meatballs to a serving dish with cranberry glaze on the side. Serve immediately. Enjoy!

20.   Wild Turkey Southwest Egg Rolls

Ingredients:

- 2 Cups Leftover Wild Turkey Meat

- 1/2 Cup Corn

- 1/2 Cup Black Beans

- 3 Tbsp Taco Seasoning

- 1/2 Cup White Onion, Chopped

- 4 Cloves Garlic, Minced

- 1 Poblano Pepper (Or 2 Jalapeño Peppers), Chopped

- 1 Can Rote Tomatoes & Chiles

- 1/2 Cup Water

- 12 Egg Roll Wrappers

Instructions:

- Add olive oil to a large skillet and heat on the stove over medium heat. Add onions and peppers and sauté

2-3 minutes until soft. Add garlic, cook 30 seconds, then Rote and black beans. Reduce heat and simmer.

- Pour taco seasoning over meat and add 1/3 cup of water and mix to coat well. Add to veggie mixture and stir to mix well. If it seems dry, add 2 tbsp water. Cook until heated all the way through.

- Remove from the heat and transfer the mixture to the fridge. The mixture should be completely cooled prior to stuffing the egg rolls or the wrappers will break.

- Place spoonful of the mixture in each wrapper and wrap tightly. Repeat with remaining wrappers. When ready to cook, set temperature to High and preheat, lid closed for 15 minutes.

- Brush each egg roll with oil or butter and place directly on the Traeger grill grate. Cook until the exterior is crispy, about 20 min per side.

- Remove from Traeger and cool. Serve. Enjoy!

21.   Smoked Wild Turkey Breast

Ingredients:

- Brine

- 2 Lbs. Turkey Breast and Deboned Thigh, Tied with Skin On

- 1 Cup Brown Sugar

- 1/4 Cup Salt

- 2 Tbsp Cracked Pepper

- 4 Cups Cold Water

- BBQ Rub

- 2 Tbsp Garlic Powder

- 2 Tbsp Onions, Dried

- 2 Tbsp Black Pepper

- 2 Tbsp Brown Sugar

- 1 Tbsp Cayenne Pepper

- 2 Tbsp Chili Powder

- 1/4 Cup Paprika

- 1 Tbsp Salt

- 2 Tbsp Sugar

- 2 Tbsp Cumin, Ground

Instructions:

- For the Brine: In a large glass bowl combine brown sugar, salt, pepper and water. Add turkey and weigh down to completely submerge if necessary. Transfer to the refrigerator and brine for 12-24 hours.

- Remove turkey from the brine and discard the brine.

- When ready to cook, set the temperature 180°F and preheat lid closed for 15 minutes.

- Combine Ingredients for the BBQ Rub. Season turkey with rub and place directly on the grill grate skin side up.

- Smoke for 5-8 hours or until the internal temperature reaches 160°F degrees when an instant read thermometer is inserted into the center.

- Remove from the smoker and let rest for 10 minutes. Turkey will continue to cook once taken off grill to reach a final temperature of 165°F in the breast.

- Slice and serve with your favorite sides. Enjoy!

22. Grilled Wild Turkey Orange Cashew Salad

Ingredients:

- Turkey Breast

- 2 Wild Turkey Breast Halves, Without Skin

- 1/4 Cup Teriyaki Sauce

- 1 Tsp Fresh Ginger

- 1 (12 Oz) Can Blood Orange Kill Cliff or Similar Citrus Soda

- 2 Tbsp Traeger Chicken Rub

- Cashew Salad

- 4 Cups Romaine Lettuce, Chopped

- 1/2 Head Red or White Cabbage, Chopped

- 1/2 Cup Shredded Carrots

- 1/2 Cup Edamame, Shelled

- 1 Smoked Yellow Bell Pepper, Sliced into Circles

- 1 Smoked Red Bell Pepper, Sliced into Circles

- 3 Chive Tips, Chopped

- 1/2 Cup Smoked Cashews

- Blood Orange Vinaigrette

- 1 Tsp Orange Zest

- Juice From 1/2 Large Orange

- 1 Tsp Finely Grated Fresh Ginger

- 2 Tbsp Seasoned Rice Vinegar

- 1 Tsp Honey

- 1/4 Cup Light Vegetable Oil

Instructions:

- For the Marinade: Combine teriyaki sauce, Kill Cliff soda and fresh ginger. Pour marinade over turkey breasts in a Ziplock bag or dish and seal. Marinate in the refrigerator for 6 to 24 hours, turning occasionally.

- When ready to cook, set temperature to 375°F and preheat, lid closed for 15 minutes.

- Remove turkey from the refrigerator, drain the marinade and pat turkey dry with paper towels.

- Place turkey into a shallow oven proof dish and season with Traeger Chicken Rub.

- Place dish in the Traeger and cook for 30-45 minutes or until the breast reaches an internal temperature of 160°F .

- Remove the breast from the grill and wrap in Traeger Butcher Paper. Let turkey rest for 10 minutes. While turkey is resting, prepare salad.

- Assemble salad Ingredients in a bowl and toss to mix. Combine all Ingredients in list for vinaigrette.

- After resting for 10 minutes, slice turkey and serve with cashew salad and blood orange vinaigrette. Enjoy!

23.   Baked Cornbread Turkey Tamale Pie

Ingredients:

- Filling

- 2 Cups Shredded Turkey

- 2 Cobs of Corn

- 1 (15 Oz) Can Black Beans, Rinsed and Drained

- 1 Yellow Bell Pepper

- 1 Orange Bell Pepper

- 2 Jalapeños

- 2 Tbsp Cilantro

- 1 Bunch Green Onions

- 1/2 Tsp Cumin

- 1/2 Tsp Paprika

- 1 (7 Oz) Can Chipotle Sauce

- 1 (15 Oz) Can Enchilada Sauce

- 1/2 Cup Shredded Cheddar Cheese

- Cornbread Topping

- 1 Cup All-Purpose Flour

- 1 Cup Yellow or White Cornmeal

- 1 Tbsp Sugar

- 2 Tsp Baking Powder

- 1/2 Tsp Salt

- 3 Tbsp Butter

- 1 Cup Buttermilk

- 1 Large Egg, Lightly Beaten

Instructions:

- For the filling: Mix to combine filling Ingredients Place in the bottom of a butter greased 10-inch pan.
- For the cornbread topping: In a mixing bowl, combine the flour, cornmeal, sugar, baking powder, and salt.

Melt the butter in a small saucepan. Remove butter from the heat and stir in the milk and egg. Make sure the mixture isn't too hot or the egg will curdle.

- Add the milk-egg mixture to the dry Ingredients and stir to combine. Do not over mix.

- To assemble Tamale Pie: Fill the bottom of a butter greased 10-inch pan with the shredded turkey filling. Top with the cornbread topping and smooth to the edges of pan.

- When ready to cook, set the temperature to 375°F and preheat, lid closed for 15 minutes.

- Place directly on the grill grate and cook for 45-50 minutes or until the cornbread is lightly browned and cooked through. Enjoy!

24.   **BBQ Pulled Turkey Sandwiches**

Ingredients:

- 6 Turkey Thighs, Skin-On

- 1 1/2 Cups Chicken or Turkey Broth

- Traeger Pork & Poultry Rub

- 1 Cup Traeger BBQ Sauce, Or More as Needed

- 6 Buns or Kaiser Rolls, Split and Buttered

Instructions:

- Season turkey thighs on both sides with the Traeger Pork & Poultry rub.
- When ready to cook, set temperature to 180°F and preheat, lid closed for 15 minutes.
- Arrange the turkey thighs directly on the grill grate and smoke for 30 minutes.
- Transfer the thighs to a sturdy disposable aluminum foil or roasting pan. Pour the broth around the thighs. Cover the pan with foil or a lid.

- Increase temperature to 325°F and preheat, lid closed. Roast the thighs until they reach an internal temperature of 180°F .

- Remove pan from the grill, but leave grill on. Let the turkey thighs cool slightly until they can be comfortably handled.

- Pour off the drippings and reserve. Remove the skin and discard.

- Pull the turkey meat into shreds with your fingers and return the meat to the roasting pan.

- Add 1 cup or more of your favorite Traeger BBQ Sauce along with some of the drippings.

- Recover the pan with foil and reheat the BBQ turkey on the Traeger for 20 to 30 minutes.

- Serve with toasted buns if desired. Enjoy!

Pork Recipes

25. Rosemary Pork Tenderloin

Preparation Time: 10 Minutes

Cooking Time: 1 hour 20 Minutes

Servings: 2

Ingredients:

- 1.5-pound pork tenderloin, fat trimmed

- 2 tablespoons minced garlic

- ¼ teaspoon ground black pepper

- 1 tablespoon Dijon mustard

- 1 tablespoon olive oil

- 6 sprigs of rosemary, fresh

Directions:

1. Open hopper of the smoker, add dry pallets, make sure ash-can is in place, then open the ash damper, power on the smoker and close the ash damper.

2. Set the temperature of the smoker to 350 degrees F, let preheat for 30 minutes, then set it to 375 degrees F and continue preheating for 20 minutes or until the green light on the dial blinks that indicate smoker has reached to set temperature.

3. Meanwhile, stir together garlic, black pepper, mustard, and oil until smooth paste comes together and then coat pork with this paste evenly.

4. Cut a kit0chen string into six 10-inch long pieces, then place them parallel to each, about 2-inch apart, lay 3 sprigs horizontally across the kitchen string, place seasoned pork on it, cover the top with remaining sprigs and tie the strings to secure the sprigs around the tenderloin.

5. Place pork on the smoker grill, shut with lid, smoke for 15 minutes, then flip the pork tenderloin and continue smoking for another 15 minutes or until the internal temperature of pork reach to 145 degrees F.

6. When done, transfer pork tenderloin to a cutting board, let rest for 5 minutes, then remove all the strong and cut pork into even slices.

Nutrition: Calories: 480 Fat: 23 g Protein: 47 g Carbs: 13 g

26.   **Pulled Pork**

Preparation Time: 25 Minutes

Cooking Time: 10 Hours And 50 Minutes

Servings: 2

Ingredients:

- 8-pound pork shoulder, fat trimmed

- 1 tablespoon garlic powder

- 1 tablespoon salt

- 1 teaspoon ground black pepper

- 1 teaspoon chipotle powder

- 1 teaspoon red chili powder

- 1 teaspoon dried thyme

- 2 tablespoons Dijon mustard

Directions:

1. Open hopper of the smoker, add dry pallets, make sure ash-can is in place, then open the ash damper, power on the smoker and close the ash damper.

2. Set the temperature of the smoker to 350 degrees F, let preheat for 30 minutes, then set it to 225 degrees F and continue preheating for 20 minutes or until the green light on the dial blinks that indicate smoker has reached to set temperature.

3. Meanwhile, rinse and pat dry pork and then coat with mustard.

4. Stir together garlic powder, salt, black pepper, chipotle powder, red chili powder, and thyme and rub this mixture on pork.

5. Place pork on the smoker grill, fat-side up, shut with lid and smoke until the internal temperature of pork reach to 160 degrees F.

6. Remove pork from the smoker and then wrap it with aluminum foil.

7. Then set the temperature of the smoker to 240 degrees F, return wrapped pork into the smoker and continue smoking the pork until the internal temperature of pork reach to 195 degrees F.

8. When you are done, transfer the pork to a cutting board, let rest for 15 minutes, then unwrap the pork and shred the meat with two forks.

9. Toss shredded pork into its juices and serve with ciabatta buns and barbecue sauce.

Nutrition: Calories: 745.8 Fat: 54.4g Protein: 53.3 g Carbs: 8.9 g

27.   Honey Glazed Ham

Preparation Time: 25 Minutes

Cooking Time: 2 Hours And 50 Minutes

Servings: 10

Ingredients:

- 8 pounds bone-in ham

- 20 whole cloves

- 1/4 cup corn syrup

- 1 cup smoked honey

- 1 stick of butter, unsalted, softened

Directions:

1. Open hopper of the smoker, add dry pallets, make sure ash-can is in place, then open the ash damper, power on the smoker and close the ash damper.

2. Set the temperature of the smoker to 350 degrees F, let preheat for 30 minutes, then set it to 325 degrees F and continue preheating for 20 minutes or until the

green light on the dial blinks that indicate smoker has reached to set temperature.

3. Meanwhile, score ham using a sharp knife, then smear the meat with butter, stuff with cloves and place ham in an aluminum foil-lined baking pan.

4. Whisk together honey and corn syrup, pour three-fourth of this mixture over ham, and then place baking pan on the smoker.

5. Shut with lid and smoke ham for 1 hour and 30 minutes or 2 hours until thoroughly cooked, and the internal temperature of ham reaches to 140 degrees F, basting ham with remaining honey mixture every 15 minutes.

6. When done, remove the pan from the grill, let rest for 15 minutes and then slice to serve.

Nutrition: Calories: 120 Fat: 5 g Protein: 16 g Carbs: 1 g

28.   Sweet & Salty Pork Belly

Preparation Time: 20 Minutes

Cooking Time: 55 Minutes

Servings:

Ingredients:

- 1-pound pork belly slices, thick-cut

- 2 teaspoons garlic powder

- 1 ½ teaspoon salt

- 1/2 cup brown sugar

- 2 teaspoons paprika

- ½ teaspoon chipotle powder

Directions:

1. Open hopper of the smoker, add dry pallets, make sure ash-can is in place, then open the ash damper, power on the smoker and close the ash damper.

2. Set the temperature of the smoker to 350 degrees F, let preheat for 30 minutes or until the green light on the

dial blinks that indicate smoker has reached to set temperature.

3. Meanwhile, place ¼ cup sugar in a shallow dish, add garlic powder, salt, paprika, chipotle pepper, stir until mixed, then rub this mixture on all sides of slices until evenly coated.

4. Place pork slices on a rimmed cookie sheet lined with aluminum foil, place it on the smoker grill, shut with lid and smoke for 10 minutes.

5. Then sprinkle the remaining sugar over pork slices and continue smoking for 15 minutes or until pork is nicely browned and sugar has caramelized.

6. When done, transfer pork belly slices to a serving dish, let cool for 10 minutes and serve.

Nutrition: Calories: 346 Fat: 43 g Protein: 29 g Carbs: 0 g

29.   Sweet Bacon Wrapped Smokes

Preparation Time: 40 Minutes

Cooking Time: 45 Minutes

Servings: 6

Ingredients:

- 14-ounce cocktail sausages

- 1-pound bacon strips, halved

- 1/2 cup brown sugar

Directions:

1. Place bacon strips on clean working space, roll them using a rolling pin until each strip is of even thickness, then wrap each strip of bacon around the sausage and secure with a toothpick.

2. Place wrapped sausages in a casserole dish in a single layer, sprinkle with sugar until covered entirely and let them rest in the refrigerator for 30 minutes.

3. Meanwhile, open hopper of the smoker, add dry pallets, make sure ash-can is in place, then open the ash

damper, power on the smoker and close the ash damper.

4. Set the temperature of the smoker to 350 degrees F, let preheat for 30 minutes or until the green light on the dial blinks that indicate smoker has reached to set temperature.

5. Lay wrapped sausage on a cookie sheet lined with parchment sheet, place the cookie sheet on the smoker grill, shut with lid and smoke for 30 minutes or until thoroughly cooked.

Nutrition: Calories: 270 Fat: 27 g Protein: 9 g Carbs: 18 g

30.   Prosciutto Wrapped Asparagus

Preparation Time: 10 Minutes

Cooking Time: 1 Hour 5 Minutes

Servings: 6

Ingredients:

- 2 bunches of asparagus

- 4-ounce prosciutto ½ tablespoon salt

- ½ tablespoon ground pepper

- 2 tablespoons apple cider vinegar, divided

- 2 tablespoons olive oil

- 3 tablespoons toasted pine nuts 1 lemon, zested

Directions:

1. Open hopper of the smoker, add dry pallets, make sure ash-can is in place, then open the ash damper, power on the smoker and close the ash damper.

2. Set the temperature of the smoker to 350 degrees F, let preheat for 30 minutes, then set it to 400 degrees F

and continue preheating for 20 minutes or until the green light on the dial blinks that indicate smoker has reached to set temperature.

3. Meanwhile, rinse asparagus, pat dry with paper towels, then cut off bottom third off of stalks and wrap 4 to 5 asparagus stalks with a piece of prosciutto.

4. Drizzle oil over asparagus bunch, drizzle with 1 tablespoon vinegar, season with salt, black pepper, and lemon zest and then place them on a baking sheet.

5. Place baking sheet on the smoker grill, then shut with lid and smoke for 5 minutes.

6. Then shake the baking pan to turn asparagus bunches, drizzle with 1 tablespoon vinegar, return the baking pan on the smoker grill and continue smoking for 5 to 8 minutes or until thoroughly cooked.

7. When done, transfer asparagus bunches to a serving dish, scatter with pine nuts and serve.

Nutrition: Calories: 56.2 Fat: 3.7 g Protein: 4 g Carbs: 2.7 g

31.   Lemon Pepper Pork Tenderloin

Preparation Time: 2 Hours And 20 Minutes

Cooking Time: 1 Hour 10 Minutes

Servings: 6

Ingredients:

- 2 pounds pork tenderloin, fat trimmed

- ½ teaspoon minced garlic 1/2 teaspoon salt

- 1/4 teaspoon ground black pepper

- 2 Lemons, zested 1 teaspoon minced parsley

- 1 teaspoon lemon juice

- 2 tablespoons olive oil

Directions:

1. Prepare the marinade and for this, place all the ingredients except for pork in a small bowl and stir until mixed.

2. Place pork tenderloin in a large plastic bag, pour in prepared marinade, seal the plastic bag, then turn it

upside down to coat the pork and marinate for a minimum of 2 hours.

3. When ready to smoke, open hopper of the smoker, add dry pallets, and make sure ash-can is in place, then open the ash damper, power on the smoker and close the ash damper.

4. Set the temperature of the smoker to 350 degrees F, let preheat for 30 minutes, then set it to 375 degrees F and continue preheating for 20 minutes or until the green light on the dial blinks that indicate smoker has reached to set temperature.

5. Remove the pork tenderloin from the marinade, place it on the smoker grill, shut with lid and smoke for 20 minutes or until thoroughly cooked and the internal temperature of pork reach to 120 degrees F; flipping pork halfway through.

6. When you are done, transfer the pork meat to a cutting board, let rest for 10 minutes, and then slice to serve.

Nutrition: Calories: 144.5 Fat: 8.8 g Protein: 13.2 g Carbs: 3.1 g

32. Bacon Wrapped Jalapeno Poppers

Preparation Time: 10 Minutes

Cooking Time: 95 Minutes

Servings: 4

Ingredients:

- 16-ounce bacon, not thick-sliced

- 10 jalapeno peppers

- 20-ounce crushed pineapple with juice

- 8-ounce cream cheese, softened

- Barbecue sauce as needed

Directions:

1. Open hopper of the smoker, add dry pallets, make sure ash-can is in place, then open the ash damper, power on the smoker and close the ash damper.

2. Set the temperature of the smoker to 350 degrees F, let preheat for 30 minutes, then set it to 275 degrees F and continue preheating for 20 minutes or until the

green light on the dial blinks that indicate smoker has reached to set temperature.

3. Meanwhile, cut each pepper lengthwise and then remove and discard its seeds.

4. Put a cream cheese in a shallow container, beat with an immersion blender until fluffy, add pineapples, mix well until combined and then stuff the mixture into jalapeno halved, leveling the top with a spatula.

5. Then wrap each stuffed jalapeno pepper with a slice of bacon and place it on a large baking sheet greased with oil; prepare the remaining wrapped peppers in the same manner.

6. Place baking sheet on the smoker grill, shut with lid and smoke for 45 minutes or until bacon is crispy.

7. Baste each pepper with a barbecue sauce and continue smoking for 5 minutes.

8. When done, transfer peppers to a dish and serve straight away.

Nutrition: Calories: 280 Fat: 26 g Protein: 9 g Carbs: 4 g

33. Pastrami

Preparation Time: 10 minutes

Cooking Time: 4-5 hours

Servings: 12

Ingredients:

- 1-gallon water, plus ½ cup

- ½ cup packed light brown sugar

- 1 (3- to 4-pound) point cut corned beef brisket with brine mix packet

- 2 tablespoons freshly ground black pepper

- ¼ cup ground coriander

Directions:

1. **Cover and refrigerate overnight, changing the water as often as you remember to do so—ideally, every 3 hours while you're awake—to soak out some of the curing salt originally added.**

2. Supply your smoker with wood pellets and follow the manufacturer's specific start-up procedure. Preheat, with the lid closed, to 275˚F.

3. In a small bowl, combine the black pepper and ground coriander to form a rub.

4. Drain the meat, pat it dry, and generously coat on all sides with the rub.

5. Place the corned beef directly on the grill, fat-side up, close the lid, and smoke for 3 hours to 3 hours 30 minutes, or until a meat thermometer inserted in the thickest part reads 175˚F to 185˚F.

6. Add the corned beef, cover tightly with aluminium foil, and smoke on the grill with the lid closed for an additional 30 minutes to 1 hour.

Remove the meat

RefrigerateNutrition: Calories: 123 Cal Fat: 4 g Carbohydrates: 3 g

Protein: 16 g Fiber: 0 g

34.   Beef Jerky

Preparation Time: 15 minutes

Cooking Time: 5 hours

Servings: 10

Ingredients:

- 3 pounds sirloin steaks

- 2 cups soy sauce

- 1 cup pineapple juice

- 1/2 cup brown sugar

- 2 tbsp. sriracha

- 2 tbsp. hoisin

- 2 tbsp. red pepper flake

- 2 tbsp. rice wine vinegar

- 2 tbsp. onion powder

Directions:

1. Mix the marinade in a zip lock bag and add the beef. Mix until well coated and remove as much air as possible.

2. Place the bag in a fridge and let marinate overnight or for 6 hours. Remove the bag from the fridge an hour prior to cooking

3. Startup the Wood Pellet and set it on the smoking settings or at 1900F.

4. Lay the meat on the grill leaving a half-inch space between the pieces. Let cool for 5 hours and turn after 2 hours.

5. Remove from the grill and let cool. Serve or refrigerate

Nutrition:

Calories: 309 Cal

Fat: 7 g

Carbohydrates: 20 g Protein: 34 g

Fiber: 1 g

35.   Smoked Beef Roast

Preparation Time: 10 minutes

Cooking Time: 6 hours

Servings: 6

Ingredients:

- · 1-3/4 pounds beef sirloin tip roast

- · 1/2 cup barbeque rub

- · 2 bottles amber beer

- · 1 bottle BBQ sauce

Directions:

1. **Turn the Wood Pellet onto the smoke setting.**

2. **Rub the beef with barbeque rub until well coated then place on the grill. Let smoke for 4 hours while flipping every 1 hour.**

3. **Transfer the beef to a pan and add the beer. The beef should be 1/2 way covered.**

4. Braise the beef until fork tender. It will take 3 hours on the stovetop and 60 minutes on the instant pot.

5. Remove the beef from the ban and reserve 1 cup of the cooking liquid.

6. Use 2 forks to shred the beef into small pieces then return to the pan with the reserved braising liquid. Add BBQ sauce and stir well then keep warm until serving. You can also reheat if it gets cold.

Nutrition:

Calories: 829 Cal

Fat: 18 g

Carbohydrates: 4 g

Protein: 86 g

Fiber: 0 g

36.   Reverse Seared Flank Steak

Preparation Time: 10 minutes

Cooking Time: 20 minutes

Servings: 2

Ingredients:

- 3 pound flank steaks

- 1 tbsp. salt

- 1/2 tbsp. onion powder

- 1/4 tbsp. garlic powder

- 1/2 black pepper, coarsely ground

Directions:

1. **Preheat the Wood Pellet to 2250F.**

2. **Add the steaks and rub them generously with the rub mixture.**

3. **Place the steak**

4. Let cook until its internal temperature is 100F under your desired temperature. 1150F for rare, 1250F for the medium rear and 1350F for medium.

5. Wrap the steak with foil and raise the grill temperature to high. Place back the steak and grill for 3 minutes on each side.

6. Pat with butter and serve when hot.

Nutrition:

Calories: 112 Cal

Fat: 5 g

Carbohydrates: 1 g

Protein: 16 g

Fiber: 0 g

37.   New York Strip

Preparation Time: 5 minutes

Cooking Time: 15 minutes Servings: 6

Ingredients:

- · 3 New York strips

- · Salt and pepper

Directions:

1. **If the steak is in the fridge, remove it 30 minutes prior to cooking.**

2. **Preheat the Wood Pellet to 4500F.**

3. **Meanwhile, season the steak generously with salt and pepper. Place it on the grill and let it cook for 5 minutes per side or until the internal temperature reaches 1280F.Rest for 10 minutes.**

Nutrition:

Calories: 198 Cal Fat: 14 g Carbohydrates: 0 g Protein: 17 g

Fiber: 0 g

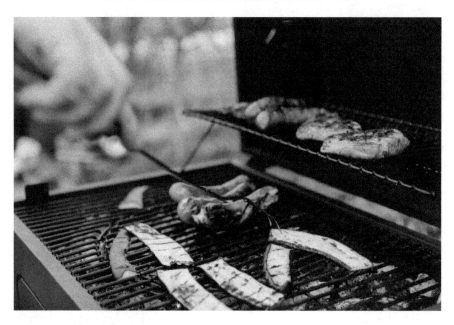

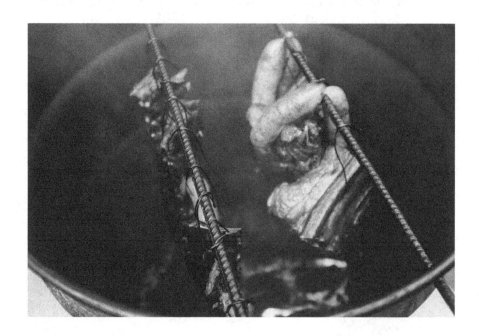

Seafood Recipes

38. Marinated Halibut Steak in Grapefruit Juice

Ingredients

- 1 Dessertspoon Freshly Chopped Marjoram

- ½ Teaspoon Salt

- 1/8 Teaspoon Freshly Ground Black Pepper

- 800grams Halibut Steaks

- 7 Tablespoons Fresh Grapefruit Juice

- 4 Tablespoons Olive Oil

- 4 Spry s Fresh Marjoram to Use as Garnish

Instructions

- In a shallow dish mix together the grapefruit juice, olive oil, freshly chopped marjoram, salt and pepper. To this mixture add the fish make sure you turn it over so both sides are coated in the marinade.

- Now cover and place in the refrigerator for 1 to 2 hours. Whilst it is marina make sure that you turn the fish over once or twice. After the marina time has elapsed you should start heat up the barbecue, with the Traeger Grill placed 4 to 6 inches above the heat source. Whilst the barbecue is heat up take the fish out of the refrigerator so that they come up to room temperature.

· When the barbecue has heated up now place the halibut steaks into a fish basket that has been lightly oiled and place on the barbecue Traeger Grill. You should cook these steaks for between 10 and 12 minutes turn them once and brush with any marinade you have left over. Serve once the steaks have become barely opaque in the thickest part on a clean plate with the sprigs of fresh marjoram.

Sauces

39.   Choran Sauce

Preparation Time: 10 minutes

Cooking Time: 30 minutes

Servings: 4

Ingredients:

- · 1 cup béarnaise sauce

- · ¼ cup tomato coulis

- · 2 tablespoons red wine vinegar

Directions:

1. **In a blender place all ingredients and blend until smooth Pour smoothie in a glass and serve**

Nutrition:

Calories 30 Fat 0g Carbs 7g Protein 0g

40.   Hot Sauce with Cilantro

Preparation Time: 10 minutes

Cooking Time: 30 minutes

Servings: 4

Ingredients:

- ½ tsp. Coriander · ½ tsp. cumin seeds · ¼ tsp. black pepper

- 2 green cardamom pods · 2 garlic cloves

- 1 tsp. Salt · 1 oz. Parsley · 2 tablespoons olive oil

Directions:

1. **In a blender place all ingredients and blend until smooth**

2. **Pour smoothie in a glass and serve**

Nutrition:

Calories: 2 Sodium: 58mg Vitamin A: 5IU Vitamin C: 0.1mg

Calcium: 1mg

CPSIA information can be obtained
at www.ICGtesting.com
Printed in the USA
BVHW011118250621
610370BV00014B/123

9 781803 016009